# Basic Stuff Series I

**volume six**

# Motor Development

**Kathleen Haywood**
University of Missouri
St. Louis, Missouri

**Thomas Loughery**
University of Missouri
St. Louis, Missouri

ISBN 0-88314-362-3

A Project of the
National Association for Sport and Physical Education
An Association of the
American Alliance for Health, Physical Education,
Recreation and Dance

# "BASIC STUFF" SERIES

A collection of booklets presenting the body of knowledge
in physical education and sport for practitioners and students.

# BASIC STUFF SERIES

**Series One**  **Informational Books**
*Patt Dodds, Series Editor*

**Exercise Physiology**
**Kinesiology**
**Motor Learning**
**Psycho-Social Aspects of Physical Education**
**Humanities in Physical Education**
**Motor Development**

**Series Two**  **Learning Experience Books**
*Norma Carr, Series Editor*

**The Basic Stuff in Action for Grades K-3**
**The Basic Stuff in Action for Grades 4-8**
**The Basic Stuff in Action for Grades 9-12**

## Editorial Committee

Elizabeth S. Bressan
University of Oregon

Norma J. Carr
SUNY, College at Cortland

Marian E. Kneer
University of Illinois, Chicago

Barbara Lockhart
University of Iowa

R. Thomas Trimble
University of Georgia

# preface

The information explosion has hit physical education. Researchers are discovering new links between exercise and human physiology. Others are investigating neurological aspects of motor control. Using computer simulation and other sophisticated techniques, biomechanics researchers are finding new ways to analyze human movement. As a result of renewed interest in social, cultural, and psychological aspects of movement, a vast, highly specialized body of knowledge has emerged.

Many physical education teachers want to use and apply information particularly relevant to their teaching. It is not an easy task. The quantity of research alone would require a dawn to dusk reading schedule. The specialized nature of the research tends to make it difficult for a layperson to comprehend fully. And finally, little work has been directed toward applying the research to the more practical concerns of teachers in the field. Thus the burgeoning body of information available to researchers and academicians has had little impact on physical education programs in the field.

The Basic Stuff series is the culmination of the National Association for Sport and Physical Education efforts to confront this problem. An attempt was made to identify basic knowledge relevant to physical education programs and to present that knowledge in a useful, readable format. The series is not concerned with physical education curriculum design, but the "basic stuff" concepts are common core information pervading any physical education course of study.

The selection of knowledge for inclusion in the series was based upon its relevance to students in physical education programs. Several common student motives or purposes for participation were identified: health (feeling good), appearance (looking good), achievement (doing better), social (getting along), aesthetic (turning on), and coping with the environment (surviving). Concepts were then selected which provided information useful to students in accomplishing these purposes.

The original Basic Stuff Series I booklets were developed to provide teachers with knowledge distilled from research in six selected disciplines which have strong implications for the ways physical educators do their work. The six disciplinary areas originally included in Series I were *Exercise Physiology, Kinesiology,* movement in the *Humanities, Psychosocial Aspects* of movement, *Motor Development,* and *Motor Learning.* The purpose of Basic Stuff Series I was to take the highly specialized knowledge and information being generated by past and current researchers and structure this knowledge (in the form of basic concepts and principles) into a simplified, readable format for efficient review and utilization.

Teams of scholars, teachers, and instructional design specialists collaborated to select the basic concepts from each discipline and to present them in appropriate form and context. Selection of knowledge was based on perceived relevance to students in physical education classes at both elementary and secondary levels of schooling. Series I was not intended to be a deliberate physical education curriculum design, or to model any sort of "ideal" or "national" curriculum, but was intended to be a resource for teachers to use in revising or developing appropriate curricula for students in their school systems.

In the revised Basic Stuff Series I, the original books were carefully reviewed, each by a small panel of scholars in that discipline. Original scholar/authors were asked to do the revisions, and five of the six agreed. The sixth book was revised by another scholar. Reviewers checked content and language of the original booklets for accuracy in restating complex ideas in simpler form, and decided whether new concepts should be added or older ones deleted or revised in light of new information available at the time of revision. The scholar/authors paid close attention to reviewers' comments as they worked to bring each book up to date to include the latest information from the discipline about which the book was written. Because the original author teams for Series I identified key concepts so thoroughly, revisions for the second edition were mostly cosmetic, involving refinement of language for clarity in expressing concepts, with a few new concepts added.

The result is a new Series designed to provide teachers at all levels with the latest information from the knowledge bases underlying effective teaching and learning of motor skills. Each book, as before, is based on concepts from a single discipline and arranged in sections referring to common student purposes for participating in movement activities. Framed as answers to questions students might ask their teachers, each concept in every booklet for a discipline is organized under the student purpose where it best fits. Student purposes for moving include HEALTH (Feeling Good), APPEARANCE (Looking Good), AESTHETICS (Turning On), COPING WITH THE ENVIRONMENT (Surviving), SOCIAL INTERACTION (Getting Along With Others), and ACHIEVEMENT (Doing Better).

Teachers may refresh their knowledge of ideas from all six disciplinary areas by reading the Series I books, then referring to Series II. The Series II books identify concepts from the various disciplines in Series I and suggest practical ways to implement them in the Physical Education setting. The Series II books are grade level specific, providing active learning experiences appropriate for Grades K-3, 4-8, and 9-12.

We hope that Basic Stuff will continue to be useful to teachers who already have discovered its merits, and that other teachers will try Basic Stuff as a potentially valuable curriculum planning resource which can help us all do our jobs better.

# table of contents

**foreword**

# foreword

Nobody needs to be reminded that kids grow! They grow, and in very much the same way their father and mother grew, their grandparents grew, and so on. With that growth, children become bigger and stronger and thus tend to improve in skill performance. But improvement in motor skills is *not* automatic. It is not the case that all children will reach a mature level of motor performance if left on their own. As Mary Ann Roberton and Lolas Halverson reveal, children who have not progressed beyond an initial skill level may enter a defeating cycle wherein they feel poorly about their skill and they avoid the opportunity to participate in activities. Their skill therefore does not develop because it is not used and they continue to feel poorly about their performance.* The challenge to those working with children is to structure environmental situations to help children develop skill. Intervention on the part of a teacher is often necessary but this intervention must be based on knowledge of growth and motor development. Even if there are few "earth shattering," new discoveries regarding physical growth, those working with children must thoroughly understand growth concepts as they form a base upon which the environment for motor development is built. Equally important to structuring that environment to help children reach their potential skill level is a thorough knowledge of the course of motor development. Children need the opportunity to understand how their growth will proceed and what skills they can expect to master at various stages of their physical growth and motor development.

*Roberton, M. A.; and Halverson, L.E., "The Developing Child — His Changing Movement." In Logsdon, B. J. et al. *Physical Education for Children.* Philadelphia, PA: Lea & Febiger, 1977, p. 63.

# health

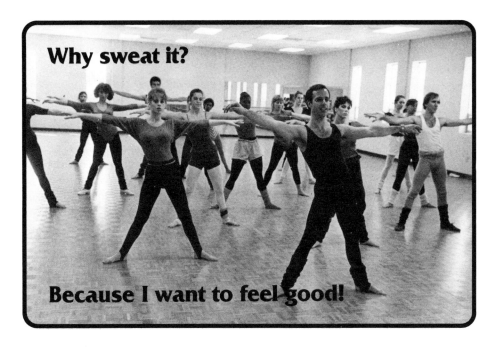

Why sweat it?

Because I want to feel good!

## What Have You Got To Help Me?

**Motor development is change in motor behavior over time**

A person's motor behavior changes over time. This change is the result of the interaction between persons and the world in which they live. It is particularly pronounced in infancy, childhood, and adolescence. How can those working with children and adolescents help them through these motor behavior changes? Certainly a thorough understanding of the changes to be expected with growth and development and the processes and influences underlying these changes can help. An understanding of motor development is essential.

For the purposes of this discussion *growth* signifies change in size; the term *development* represents changes in function. More specifically motor development relates to maturation of the neuromuscular mechanism which permits progressive performance in motor skills.

It is desirable for these changes to lead to the optimal level of performance each individual can achieve. Change to the most efficient motor behavior does not automatically come with time. Nor are certain accomplishments guaranteed when one matures to a given age. One need only observe the motor behavior of most adults to know that! Help and intervention is necessary for most persons to achieve better motor performance. This help must be purposeful, based on a knowledge of what critical aspects of skill performance to observe, what changes are possible, and what environmental structuring will assist change.

**Children often move for joy**

Why be concerned with helping others achieve better motor performance? It feels good to carry out a skill successfully and efficiently! People enjoy doing a skill well because it means they can usually accomplish the most for the least energy expended. Consider running as an example. Running can be an excellent activity for improving the fitness of children and adults alike. Young children often have a running form in which they swing their legs to the side rather than bringing them directly forward. Energy appears to be wasted on unnecessary movement. Thus there is less energy to continue running and maximize the health and fitness benefits of the activity. Young children, however, are practicing emerging skills, all of which appear in an immature form. Often the joy of movement is a function of the harmony between body parts in executing a skill for goal achievement. Young children often move for the sheer joy of moving.

With more effective motor performance also comes increasing opportunities to engage in physical activities. When the basic motor skills can be performed well they can be used in learning new and more complex forms of play, games, or dances. More emphasis can be placed on meeting increasingly difficult challenges. Broader and more varied opportunities to engage in healthful activity will also increase the likelihood that an individual will participate in some kind of physical activity throughout their life span. More skillful motor performance makes activity more challenging and enjoyable!

## Why Does It Happen That Way?

**Motor development reflects changes in a person and changes in how they interact with their environment**

The motor behavior changes occurring with time reflect the interaction between persons and the world in which they live. Specifically these changes represent the reciprocal relationships between growth and development. During childhood and adolescence there are many changes in the

2

body including increases in height and weight, changes in the body proportions and in body composition, and so on. To understand why the motor behavior changes occur in certain ways during childhood and adolescence one must understand the relationship between physical growth and development. In addition, growth and development changes may be confusing and mysterious to the young performer. Helping youth understand growth and development, what changes to expect in their body, what changes are genetically controlled, and what changes are environmentally influenced, also helps them set appropriate goals and realize success.

**Activities should be appropriate to the developmental level**

An understanding of physical growth and development is also the basis on which one can structure the environment for motor performance. Thus activities can be changed to accomodate size variations among children of the same age, differences in muscle strength, differences in limb proportions, and differences in developmental levels. Boundaries of games may be changed, the size of equipment used in certain activities changed, rule adaptations made, and the number and roles of the participants varied. These variations can then be based on knowledge of growth and development and the interaction between the growing body and the environment.

A second aspect of changing motor behavior is the changing process of perception. There are predictable changes in the ways in which children perceive and interpret the world around them. Naturally these changes affect the motor behavior made in response to the environment.

There are many, many other ways in which the person interacts with the world to influence changes in motor behavior. Many will be discussed in the questions and answers that follow. Others will be discussed in other "Basic Stuff" booklets. Those who appreciate why these interactions influence changes in motor behavior can better assist young performers to first understand the changes in their behavior and then make a smooth transition through these changes to a high level of skill . . . and that FEELS GOOD!

# appearance

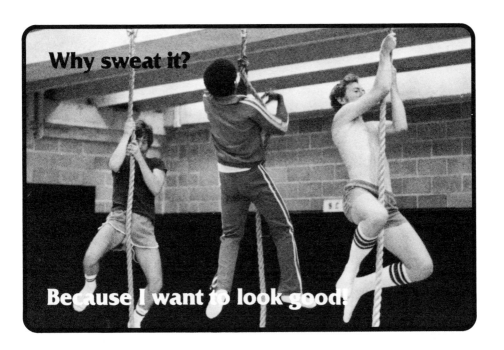

Why sweat it?

Because I want to look good!

## What Do You Have To Help Me?

**Growth patterns affect appearance**

Shortly after the birth of a child, mothers and fathers proudly accept compliments from friends and relatives regarding the appearance of the newborn, such as, "My, what a cute baby!" From this point on, the physical appearance of the growing child is important to the parents and relatives. Young children soon learn the cultural and societal importance of a pleasing appearance. The child who presents a pleasant appearance indicated by facial and selected body features may reap more social rewards such as acceptance by others than does the child who presents a less than pleasing physical appearance. This does not mean that beauty is the most cherished or important personal possession but that children soon learn certain positive and negative effects of appearance.

5

While it is commonly understood that physical appearance is strongly based on genetic factors, there are many indications that certain aspects are based on environmental factors. Some of the major physical factors that are influenced by genes are height, length of limbs, and facial features. The potential for the growth of the bones, limbs, and trunk are established at conception. The pattern of growth is also indicated by genetic factors. In many cases some phases of the growth and development pattern may be rapid in certain individuals and slow in others. This affects one's relationship to a group since a child might be a head taller than any of the other children in a class.

Growth patterns that can be controlled by environmental factors generally include body composition and posture. Body composition in this instance refers to the ratio of lean or fat-free weight to fat weight. Many recent studies indicate that the nutritional and exercise habits developed in infancy have an effect on such habits later in life. Those who eat poorly and rarely exercise in childhood often maintain these habits throughout life and thus maintain a body composition high in fat weight and low in fat-free weight. Yet body composition can be and is of great concern especially to school age children because it greatly influences peer acceptance and self-concept. For instance the obese child who faces negative comments from classmates about physical size not only endures such forms of rejection but also has to personally deal with the limitations an obese body type places on participation in some physical activities. Even the "skinny" child may face derogatory comments from peers. Although not faced with the same physical limitations the slender child may not have as much physical strength or endurance as other children.

# How Do I Get It?

As a person matures, the most noticeable change is found in physical size; children become taller and heavier. There are other less obvious ways the body changes. The relative lengths of the arms, legs, and trunk change. The bones are growing as is the muscle tissue. The amounts of fat tissue and fat-free tissue in the body can also change as a child grows and develops. All of these changes may affect participation in physical activity. The extent to which one is active may in turn affect body appearance.

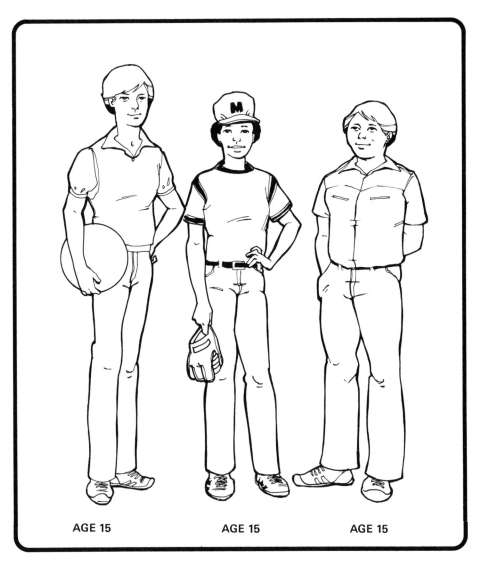

**AGE 15**          **AGE 15**          **AGE 15**

Growth patterns can affect relationships with peers.

The body also changes in a way not outwardly visible. This is the basis for motor development. The nervous system which controls body functions, thinking, and physical movements, increases in complexity. While babies are born with the greatest number of nerve cells they will ever have, the number of connections each cell makes with other nerve cells increases throughout childhood and into adolescence. The amount of myelin around some parts of the nerve cell also increases through adolescence and this change promotes the speed and integrity of nerve signals. These changes affect one's potential skill in physical activities. Skilled actions are determined through the processes of perceiving the goal to be attained, making decisions concerning the body response to the task, and then carrying out the response. How these factors change as one grows and which factors can be altered will be discussed in the following pages.

# How?

**Growth occurs in
definite patterns**

Growth and development follow definite patterns. This pattern is illustrated in Figure 1. These patterns begin with very rapid growth from birth to two years of age followed by a period of consistent, stable growth until 8 or 9 years. Some time after this boys and girls enter a period of very rapid growth sometimes referred to as the "adolescent growth spurt." The peak rate of growth comes on the average at 12 years of age for girls and 14 years of age for boys. After this peak, growth continues for at least 2 or 3 more years before stopping.

**Individual growth
rates vary**

Although people follow the same general growth pattern, they have their own timing. Some children will be a year or two ahead of the average maturity level for their age while others may be a year or two behind. If one could X-ray the growing bones of each child, the level of skeletal maturation would be known. Since this isn't advisable it is useful to know that body size is closely related to maturation. For example taller and heavier children tend to be early maturers while shorter and lighter children tend to be late maturers. Individual differences in maturation rates are present in preadolescence but the differences are highlighted when some enter the adolescent growth spurt and achieve sexual maturation at an earlier age than others.

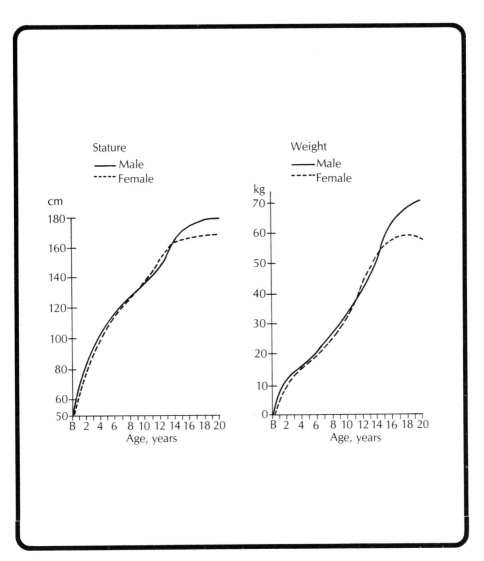

**Figure 1: Distance curves for height, showing the adolescent spurt of males and females.**
From R. Malina, *Growth and Development: The First Twenty Years In Man* (Minneapolis Burgess, 1975), p. 19.

At birth some parts of the body are closer to adult size than other parts. The head, for example, is approximately one-half its adult size but the legs are only one-fifth of their adult length. Some parts of the body must grow faster than other parts during childhood and adolescence to reach adult proportions, as shown in Figure 2. Of the body areas, the arms and legs grow the fastest between one year and puberty while the trunk grows most rapidly between puberty and mature stature.

There is very little difference in height and weight between girls and boys until girls enter the adolescent growth spurt. Girls usually begin their growth spurt between ten and one-half and thirteen years while boys begin their spurt between twelve and one-half and fifteen years. For several years girls may be taller than boys of the same age. At all ages the inter-sex differences are more noticeable than the intra-sex differences. Between the ages of thirteen and fifteen, boys generally pass the girls and will be, on the average, taller and heavier. The average boy is five feet nine and one-half inches tall and one hundred fifty two pounds by age eighteen while the average girl is five feet four and one-half inches tall and one hundred twenty five pounds.

Height is basically
determined by genetic
factors
No one can predict exactly how tall a child will be but height is greatly influenced by the genes received from one's parents. Parents pass on a "growth potential" or the probability of achieving a certain height. Whether or not one reaches this height is influenced by environmental factors which include nutrition and disease. A child of short parents will most likely be shorter than average and a child of tall parents will most likely be taller than average. While growth potential cannot be changed, good health and nutrition can be maintained.

# What Else?

Mild exercise stress
stimulates bone
strength and growth
How do bones change during growth? Even though they are thought of as being hard the bones are really changing all the time. Throughout life new cells are constantly replacing old ones. When one is young and growing taller there are parts of the bones where new cells are laid down and calcified to increase the length of the long bones or the size of small, round bones. The blood supply to the bones is necessary for maintenance of normal bone strength and bone growth. Exercise which induces mild stress improves circulation of the

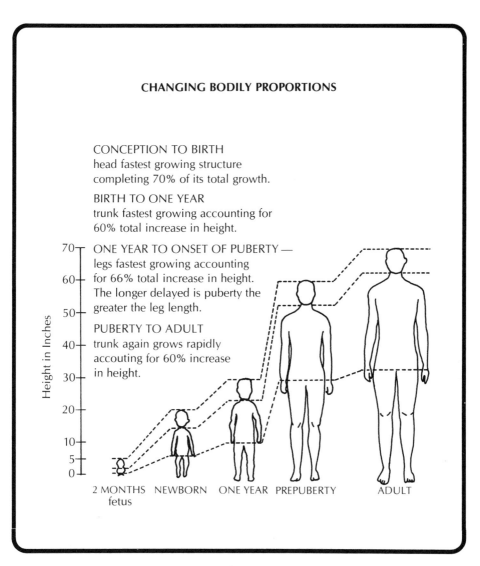

**Figure 2: Changing body proportions from conception to adulthood.** From D. Whipple, *Dynamics of Development: Euthenic Pediatrics.* (New York: McGraw-Hill, 1966), p. 122. Used with permission of McGraw-Hill.

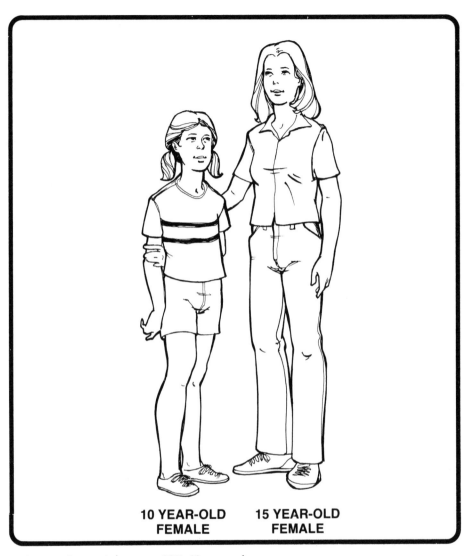

**10 YEAR-OLD FEMALE**     **15 YEAR-OLD FEMALE**

Girls' growth spurt is between 10½-13 years of age.

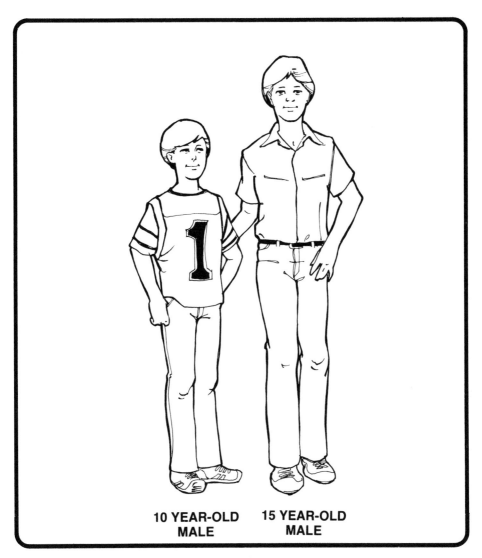

**10 YEAR-OLD MALE**     **15 YEAR-OLD MALE**

Boys' growth spurt is between 12½-15 years of age.

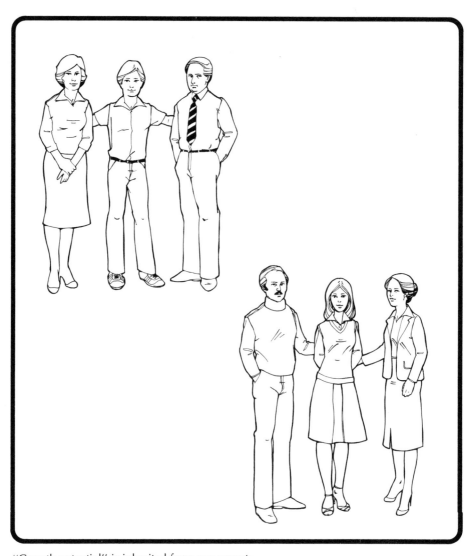

"Growth potential" is inherited from our parents.

blood and influences bone strength and growth. On the other hand some activities put severe stress on the part of a bone where growth is occurring and may cause an injury to that area. One example of this comes in baseball; constantly attempting to throw a curve ball at a young age can injure the part of the upper arm bone near the elbow where some forearm muscle tendons attach to the bone. Some of these bone injuries may result in a disturbance of or even premature cessation of bone growth. Different bones stop growing at different ages. Once they stop and the center for laying down new cells no longer functions the bone will no longer grow. Once growth in the length and size of bones has stopped in late adolescence it cannot be started again.

# What Else?

**Muscle growth parallels general body growth**

What about muscle growth? Muscle growth follows the same pattern as general body growth. After a rapid growth of muscle mass during the first two years there is a gradual, stable gain in muscle mass consistent with general body growth during childhood and pre-adolescence. This growth occurs through an increase in the size rather than the number of cells. Although boys have slightly higher estimates of lean body mass, or fat-free weight, the muscular differences between boys and girls before puberty are minimal. During adolescence boys experience a substantial increase in lean or fat-free weight largely due to an increase in muscle mass. Girls, on the other hand, experience a much smaller increase in lean or fat-free weight. By adulthood the average woman will have two-thirds of the fat-free body weight of the average male.

# How Do I Get It?

**Muscle size is influenced by the sex hormones and exercise**

Can the size of the muscles be increased? As previously discussed the muscle cells increase in size as one grows. Muscles also respond to exercise by increasing in mass. This size increase is relatively small unless a hormone called testosterone is present in the body. In boys, testosterone is first produced in large quantities at the onset of adolescence. Pre-adolescent boys and girls and women do not have testosterone levels high enough to bring about a large increase in the size of their muscles with exercise. This does not mean they cannot increase the strength of their muscles because a

15

muscle needn't be dramatically increased in size to increase strength. During adolescence and adulthood men can undertake certain kinds of training programs which may greatly increase the size of the muscles.*

# What Else?

Fat content is
influenced by eating
habits and exercise

The fat content of the body also influences appearance. Aside from a very small percentage of people with certain medical problems one controls the amount of fat weight in his body. This is accomplished by tracking the number of calories taken in and the number expended to maintain the body and carry out activities. If these are balanced, body weight is maintained. If one eats more than one uses, weight is gained. Growing boys and girls need to eat enough calories for their bodies to support the growth of new tissues as well as carry out normal body functions and activities. As one grows older and growth slows down fewer calories are needed for building new body tissues. The caloric needs *per pound* of body weight decrease. For example, the calories needed daily per pound of body weight decreases from 35 at age 4 years, to 28 at age 8, to 23 at age 12, and to 20 by adulthood. The *total* number of calories needed might rise because the body weight increases with growth. An 8-year-old girl weighing 75 pounds needs approximately 2100 calories per day, while a 12-year-old girl weighing 75 pounds needs approximately 1725 calories per day. Yet, a 12-year-old weighing 100 pounds needs approximately 2300 calories per day.

As the body grows and increases in size, the amount of fat one has increases. These increases are marked during the first year and following ages 6 to 8 years. During adolescence the hormone estrogen promotes the accumulation of fat in girls. This accumulation is greatest in the hips, buttocks, breasts and inner calves. Boys do not accumulate as much fat as girls during adolescence and it may be differently distributed. For example adolescent boys usually show an increase in the thickness of fat near their shoulder blades but a decrease in the upper arm.

Everyone's body has some fat weight and it is necessary to balance exercise and caloric intake so that the proportion of

*Further information on muscle strength development may be found in the "Basic Stuff" booklet on Exercise Physiology.

fat weight doesn't become too high. Exercise is very important in controlling the fat weight of the body. It promotes the amount of fat-free weight at the expense of fat.

# Why Does It Happen That Way?

**Growth generally improves physical ability**

The body changes that occur prior to maturity can either be beneficial to participation in physical activity or can be detrimental to participation. In most instances skill will be improved through the increase in body size and strength and neuromuscular development. However it is possible for performance level to decrease as one grows. This might happen if the number of calories eaten is greater than the number used and excess body fat is accumulated or it may happen if one fails to regularly stretch the muscles and thus lose joint flexibility.

**Performance quality is influenced by maturity and experience**

The number of physical activities in which a mature person will be able to participate successfully should be much greater than those of a small child. The performance quality should increase not only to the point of maturity but for many years thereafter due to increased performing experience. There are other reasons for the increase in the quantity and quality of physical performance to the point of physical maturity and beyond. Some of the reasons may be related to the opportunities for participation available to developing children. Included in these opportunities would be such factors as play and recreation equipment available at home, school, or in the community, motivation of the child and parents to participate in physical activity, interests and expertise of physical education teachers and sports instructors, and time and money available for participation.

**Growth in height and weight alters the mechanical nature of physical performance**

In addition to these factors relating to opportunities for participation one must consider the factors relating to physical development. Physical development includes growth, neuromuscular maturation, and perceptual and sensory development. Successful participation in some physical activities is greatly enhanced by increased physical size. In other words a larger person would be able to perform some activities better than a smaller person. A person who is six feet tall should be capable of performing much better than a person who is four feet tall in a high jump event in terms of their absolute jump height. Growth in height and weight alters the mechanical nature of physical performance. The larger person has longer limbs, more range of motion, and larger muscles. Little success can be expected in shooting baskets at a regulation ten-foot goal until the person is tall enough and strong enough to propel a regulation ball high enough to score. In other activities a small body size may be more desirable than a larger one. Just consider gymnastics where both men and women who excel in world-wide competition are shorter in height than the average for their age.

**Perceptual and sensory development increases performance effectiveness**

As physical growth and development occurs gradually and steadily, so does perceptual and sensory development. Such factors as visual discrimination, distinguishing visual stimuli, visual tracking, and following a moving stimulus are vitally important in most activities. In many activities the stimuli are in constant or nearly constant motion and the participant or participants constantly need to alter their positions to interact successfully with the stimuli. Participation in the game of soccer involves 22 players and one ball that may all be in simultaneous motion. The players must make split-second decisions regarding their relationship to the ball and to other players to determine what is the proper skill and strategy to use at that particular moment. With maturation of the nervous system, increasingly complex situations may be judged so that the best response may be selected and carried out. Perceptual and sensory development and decision-making are factors in the increasing ability to perform physical activities with increased effectiveness.

# How?

**Mature appearance is influenced by genetic and environmental factors**

Some of our body features are determined by the genes inherited from our parents and little can be done to change them. Among these are body height, the length of the limbs, color of the hair and eyes, and facial structure. One also tends to have a body build or shape determined by heredity. On the other hand there are things about the body which reflect the exercise one obtains through activities. If one is active there is a tendency to have more fat-free weight and less fat weight in the body. In other words body composition reflects activity level.

There are differences in body shapes between males and females especially after the onset of adolescence. Many of these have been brought about by the different hormones manufactured by boys' and girls' bodies. Boys start their growth spurt later but it lasts longer. The growth centers in

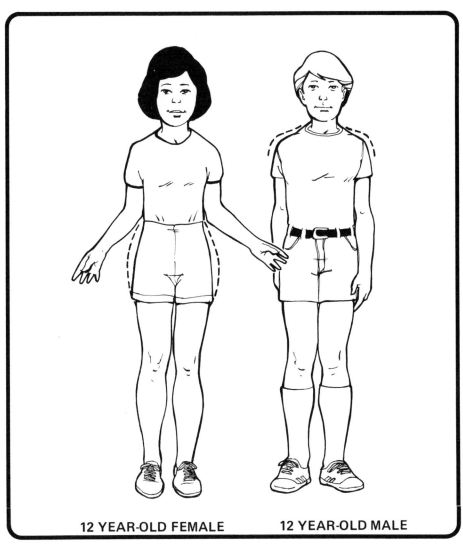

**12 YEAR-OLD FEMALE**     **12 YEAR-OLD MALE**

During adolescence, boys increase in shoulder width and girls increase in hip width.

their bones are active over a longer period of time and on the average, men are taller than women. They also have relatively longer legs than women. In adolescence, boys also increase in shoulder width while their hip width remains relatively narrow. Girls, on the other hand, increase in hip width. As mentioned before, girls add some fat tissue to the hips, breasts, buttocks, and inner calves. This is just enough tissue to give a girl a woman's "figure" and there isn't a great deal of fat if she eats sensibly and exercises. Boys have a marked increase in fat-free weight during adolescence while girls experience a much smaller increase in fat-free weight.

# How Do I Get It?

**Physical activity and exercise may improve appearance**

Can one improve appearance? The answer to this has to be an equivocal yes and no. As was discussed earlier, certain genetic factors influence one's appearance at maturity. Yet there are environmental factors that determine to some extent what one will look like at maturity. The genetic factors are determined at conception and generally cannot be altered but the environmental factors can be changed. How one looks at maturity and thereafter is also influenced by environmental factors.

Such physical characteristics as height, body proportion, and facial appearance are determined by genetic factors and cannot be easily altered for appearance improvement. Other physical characteristics such as muscular development and body composition can be altered. Physical activity is one of the factors that is the most significant in bringing about such desired changes. Nutrition and diet are other important factors. When proper nutrition and proper diet is combined with the proper type and amount of physical activity the muscular development and body composition can be greatly enhanced. Corrective exercises can improve the posture of an individual through the strengthening of certain muscles and the stretching of other muscles. These concepts are discussed in more detail in later sections of this book and in other books of this series.

# achievement

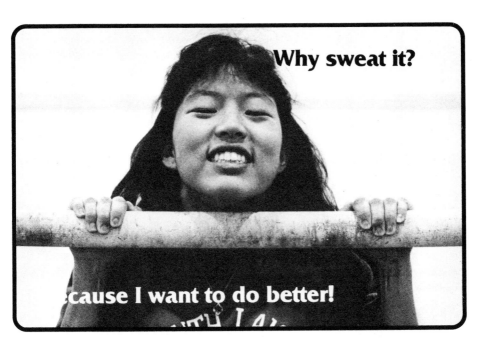

**Why sweat it?**

**cause I want to do better!**

## What Have You Got To Help Me?

**Basic skills are fundamental to successful participation**

If one looks at the popular sports, games, or dances it is apparent that all of the complex movements used are combinations of *basic skills*. Examine basketball. During a basketball game, players will probably run, jump, turn, bend, throw, and strike. They may do these things in many ways, not doing the exact same thing twice. The players in trying to accomplish a goal are performing movements made up of their basic skills "vocabulary." To enjoy activities like games, sports, and dance, one must learn basic skills.

Many things including fitness, instruction, and practice are necessary to develop good basic skills. Between the ages of two and seven, children generally improve their basic skills by developing changes in their *form* among other ways. It may be that everyone goes through stages in developing

21

mature skills. There may be stages for different body areas like arm action, trunk action, or leg action. Some people pass through one stage very quickly while others spend a long time performing a skill at one stage level. Whether or not we all go through definable stages in acquiring mature skills, there appear to be trends which occur with advancing age which are consistent with sound mechanical principles (see "Efficient Use of Force in Basic Skills" in Chapter 1 of the Kinesiology book in this series). As mature throwing skills are acquired, performers improve in their ability to use both linear (straight line) motion as with a step forward, and rotational motion as the twisting of the trunk. It is important to understand the mechanical principles related to movement because with understanding, "doing better" in basic and complex skills is possible.

# How Do I Get It?

**Complex skills are comprised of the basic skills of locomotion, nonlocomotion and manipulation, and perceptual-motor responses.**

Just what are the basic skills? There are so many different types of physical activities in which people can participate. Some activities require a great deal of movement and involve the total body whereas some activities require little movement and involve only certain body parts and muscle groups. Here the emphasis will be placed on developing skill in a wide range of physical activities.

Many systems have been devised to classify physical activities on the basis of the type of movement involved. In every case the activities have been classified primarily on the basis of the complexity of the movement or movement combinations. Such classification systems reflect the developmental factors associated with successful participation in physical activity. The mastery of certain basic movements is necessary before more complex skills and patterns of movement can be learned.

**Basic skills are the foundation for complex skills**

Generally fundamental movement patterns can be classified into four categories: locomotor skills; non-locomotor skills; manipulative skills; perceptual-motor skills. The locomotor skills are those skills such as walking, running, galloping, etc. that enable us to move from one place to another. The non-locomotor skills are those skills such as bending, pushing, stretching, etc. that are done in a relatively stationary position with little or no movement from one place to another. The manipulative skills are those skills such as kicking, throwing, striking, etc. an object from one place to another either as one is moving or in a stationary position. The perceptual motor skills are skills requiring coordination, form perception, spatial awareness, etc. that help a performer perceive and react to various forms and objects that are involved in many activities. While it is possible to place movements and skills into such categories one must remember that a combination of each of these movements and skills are generally involved in games and activities.

As children grow and develop they should be able to successfully participate in more complex patterns of movements and games. The newborn infant is generally incapable of engaging in locomotor movement in the first few months of life but is capable of performing simple non-locomotor movements such as twisting, stretching, etc. Basic forms of locomotor movement may be mastered by the age of two while more complex forms of locomotor movement such as leaping and skipping may not be mastered until the child approaches eight to ten years of age. Perceptual-motor skills such as balance also follow a definite developmental pattern that is closely related to perceptual development factors. Before refinement of complex physical skills can be accomplished, visual perception, depth perception, auditory perception, tactile perception, and kinesthetic awareness need to be developed. In manipulative activities such as catching and throwing, successful participation is dependent upon the development of perceptual motor factors. A small child can kick a stationary ball but may not be capable of successfully kicking a moving ball.

Higher level or more complex games—games that involve many different types of skills—cannot be mastered until one has developed the basic skills and movement patterns that are a part of that particular game. That is why the physical education program emphasizes basic locomotor, non-locomotor, and perceptual motor skills during the early school years. By doing so the basic skills can be developed which are essential for successful participation in a wide variety of activities. As children develop and master these basic skills they are then prepared for more complex skills that involve a combination of each of these basic skills.

# How Else Do I Get It?

**Perception affects
motor responses**

Motor responses always involve the processing of sensory and perceptual information by the central nervous system. Sensory receptors first establish information about the environment and one's position in it. These "afferent" signals are relayed to the central nervous system where they are evaluated, interpreted, and compared to previous experiences. This process is called "perception." Sensory and perceptual information is necessary before one can select and plan a motor response and send an "efferent" signal to the muscles to carry out the response. If one can process the afferent information quickly and precisely, motor behavior will be skillful. Development of more and more complex perceptual motor responses occurs as a child can process more and more complex information about the environment. This gives a child a greater potential for control of visible motor responses.

## Why Does It Happen That Way?

**Changes occur in perceptual processing**

There are three processes in which perceptual motor development occurs. First a child shifts from a dominance of internal tactile and kinesthetic sensory receptors to dominance of receptors (especially the eyes) soliciting information from the environment. Early in life children rely heavily on what they feel through the tactile receptors. Later they can plan and execute responses based on visual information with accuracy. For example one can teach a very young child to assume a batting stance and to execute a swing. The child's accuracy in hitting the ball, however, is related to the pitcher's accuracy in throwing where the child will swing not just the child's ability to judge where the ball will be! Later a child will be able to concentrate on the ball, i.e., gather visual information, and coordinate a response to it.

Secondly children will improve in their ability to integrate the afferent signals from two or more receptors in different systems. Visual information will be matched with a sound, a sound with the feel of an object, and so on. Rather than responding to the signals from just one system, children will increasingly be able to make use of multiple signals from multiple systems. Visual information about a bat striking a ball will be matched with the sound of the event and a motor response may be executed based on both input signals.

Finally, children develop an increasing capacity to differentiate cues within a system. They detect smaller differences between two signals or smaller similarities in them. They may discriminate between the kinesthetic feel which sends a ball to the right of a target and the one which sends it directly to the target.

The shift to visual system dominance has typically occurred in children by seven or eight years. Improved intersensory communication and intrasensory discrimination seems to develop simultaneously. The biggest improvement in these areas also comes between three and six years of age but is related to the child's previous experience with tasks which makes demands on the visual system. Thus children differ in their levels of intersensory communication and intrasensory discrimination. A slowly developing child is likely to demonstrate deficits in these processes when compared to a normally developing child. This may lead to more difficulty on the part of the slowly developing child to perform motor tasks.

# What Have You Got To Help Me?

**Skilled performance discriminations are based on perceptual information**

The perceptual discriminations needed for skilled performance are varied and arise from many types of sensory receptors. The brain processes information sensed by the eyes which influence judgments about depth, color, form, relative size, object constancy, and figures against a background. To accurately make these judgements one must have at least minimal levels of visual acuity, peripheral vision, and ocular tracking. Sensory receptors in the inner ear provide information about balance and orientation in space. Those in the joints including the neck, tendons, muscles, and skin contribute to kinesthetic awareness and a sense of how the body parts are positioned. The signals from these receptors give rise to a sense of laterality (distinguishing the left and right sides of the body), directionality (projecting left and right into space), and body image. Discriminations about sounds are also important as are those about objects which are touched.

**Performance is enhanced by sharpness of sight**

To make judgments about moving objects or judgments concerning one's body moving in relation to fixed objects, objects must be brought into sharp focus. Visual acuity refers to the sharpness of vision or the extent to which one can discriminate fine detail. A "Snellen score" is typically used to describe the level of acuity with 20/20 vision being acceptable. Children by five years of age have approximately 20/30 vision. Visual acuity of 20/20 is not reached until about 7 years of age because the eyeball tends to be relatively short front-to-back and vision is therefore farsighted, meaning near objects are not clearly seen.

Although the need to see objects sharply is important to skilled performance there are other visual abilities required as well. One of these is the perception of depth which depends on visual acuity, coordinated use of the two eyes, and fusion or the ability of the brain to merge the images seen by each eye. At least gross levels of depth perception are present in the first months of life. Children at about 6 years are fairly accomplished in depth perception because visual acuity is close to adult levels and fusion, the merging of images seen by each eye into one, occurs at about this age.

It is also important in movement activities to track or pursue a moving object with the eyes. These movements, whether they precisely follow an object or allow brief periods of fixation of a moving object project the object's image onto the section of the eye's retina yielding the most acuity. Newborn infants can track an object but their eye movements are not very precise. Pursuit tracking becomes more precise throughout childhood and probably improves into early adolescence. Most children at eight years of age are certainly capable of accurate judgments about moving objects.

Little perception of color is evident in the newborn. Children at 3 and 4 years may still prefer shape to color as a way of classifying objects. By 6 years of age color is used extensively to discriminate objects. While the importance of color perception to motor skills is unclear some color combinations of moving objects against backgrounds have been shown to yield better catching in children than other combinations. These combinations may assist a child's figure-ground perception, or ability to identify the object of interest against a background.

In dealing with objects in physical space, one must perceive that objects maintain a constant size despite the fact that their distance from the observer varies. As distance varies the object takes up more or less space on the observer's retina in the rear of the eye. This type of perception is called size constancy. Young children often make errors in judging sizes and distances. In particular they tend to overestimate the distance between two objects or people as they get farther and farther away. The perception of size constancy approaches adult levels by approximately 11 years of age.

An object of visual interest is often embedded in a distracting background. One must locate and focus on the object, ignoring the background. This is often true in skills wherein one must catch or strike an approaching ball. This perception of figure-and-ground improves in spurts, one between 4 and 6 years of age and another between 6 and 8 years of age with near-adult levels shown thereafter (Williams, 1983). Young children find it easier to locate objects with which they are familiar.

Another aspect of visual perception is the ability to discriminate parts of an object from the whole. For example, one with refined whole-part perception could recognize a clown assembled from pieces of candy as just that, but a young child might report seeing just the clown or just the candy. By the age of approximately 9, children can integrate parts and the whole.

An object's orientation or arrangement in space is important. Sometimes one must ignore orientation, as in recognizing which base is first base whether one is in the field or at bat. At other times differences in orientation are critical, as is the case in reading "d" and "b". Young children learn to attend to spatial orientation before they can ignore it, often thinking two like objects are different if they are oriented differently. Children of 3 and 4 years can appreciate orientations along vertical and horizontal but many cannot differentiate obliques and diagonals until approximately 8.

Between the ages of 3 and 5 nearly all children show eye dominance. That is one eye tends to lead the other in fixation (maintaining gaze on an object). Eye dominance is usually maintained throughout life once it is established. While there is some thought that performers whose dominant eye is on the same side as their dominant hand have an advantage in some skills many "cross-laterals" perform skills quite well.

Since most of the information about the skilled tasks one undertakes comes from the visual system, visual perception is critical to skilled activities. Children need to have their eyes periodically examined so that correctable deficits in eye function may be detected. Those with normal vision who have deficits in visual perception may need remedial activities before achieving success in many skills.

# What Else Have You Got To Help Me?

**Knowing the position of the body in space is necessary for skill performance**

While vision is important to skilled performance it is also necessary to know the location of the body and its parts in space. This information comes from many sources. Signals from the receptors in the inner ear, along with vision, help one achieve and maintain balance. Receptors in the head and neck keep the head upright when it needs to be. One can determine the location of arms, legs, and trunk through signals from receptors in the skin, joints, muscles, and tendons. All of these signals contribute to one's *kinesthetic awareness*. As one becomes aware of the body and how it can be used, body image or self-concept is developed (because the position of the body in relation to objects and its parts is perceived). This gives one confidence as new skills or new combinations of old skills are attempted.

The receptors in the skin, joints, muscles, and tendons function quite early in life. As discussed earlier one improves in matching kinesthetic information with that from the other senses and in discriminating kinesthetic information during childhood and early adolescence. Varied movement experiences contribute to the development of perceptions of the body and its place in space; this represents improved kinesthetic awareness. On the other hand slowly developing children are typically dependent upon visual information for their awareness of space. Their spatial awareness appears to come from one sense rather than the integrating of information from the various senses with kinesthetic receptors. Therefore less information is available or the information is contradictory and the exact position of the body in space is not accurately perceived.

There are several aspects of body awareness. Children must become aware that their body and its parts are a part of themselves and not the environment; they recognize that a body part can be moved and positions imitated even before they attach verbal labels to the body parts. By five or six years most children can name the major body parts and by eight or nine few mistakes are made in naming them. Another aspect of body awareness is laterality, or an awareness that the body has two distinct sides. This awareness may also precede one's ability to label the sides "right" and "left." By four years of age most children have established a preferential use of one of the hands or feet. For several years after this, however, a child may show ambivalence in hand use until dominance is firmly established by age nine or ten. About age nine, children can consistently label the sides and body parts "right" and "left." Closely related to laterality is the perception of "up and down" and "front and back" within the body. Although evidence is lacking many believe these concepts are realized slightly before laterality is established. Naturally the ability to label body parts and to establish dominance is important to functioning in the world as well as to the ability to perform skills.

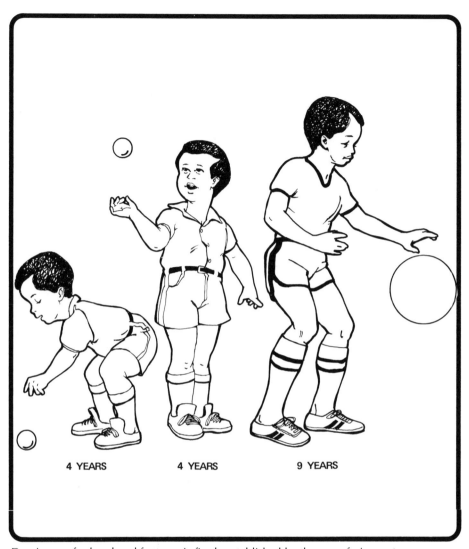

4 YEARS     4 YEARS     9 YEARS

Dominance for hand and foot use is firmly established by the age of nine or ten.

**Development of body awareness, balance, spatial awareness, and tactile location aids performance**

Whether body awareness forms the basis for spatial awareness or simply precedes it in development is unclear but spatial awareness is certainly important to movement in space. One must be able to perceive relationships between one's own body and objects or places in space. These include directions such as right, left, up, down, forward, backward, etc., and relationships such as "in front of," "behind," "next to," and so on. It would certainly be difficult to learn to dance or perform an offensive play in basketball without a sense of spatial awareness! Children benefit from undertaking a variety of tasks meant to establish relationships between their body and other objects.

Balance is also an important part of performing skills. While the receptors for balance information are mature after several years of life, improvement on a variety of balance tasks seems to come through childhood and on some tasks into adolescence. This improvement may reflect increasing ability to discriminate information from the balance receptors; it represents increased strength. Balance tasks are also helpful to children and a variety of tasks will give them many chances to discriminate and interpret information from the balance receptors as well as chances to make corrections of their body position based on this information (because there is little evidence of a generalized balance ability). It is important to give children many types of balance experiences. One who performs a given balance task well may not necessarily be able to perform another balance task well.

Identifying a spot or touch on the body (without vision) is an aspect of kinesthetic awareness. So too, is the ability to discriminate two separate touches in the same body area. Children of approximately 5 years of age can identify one touch but have difficulty discriminating touches on different fingers. The latter ability improves through at least 7 1/2 years.

# What Else?

**Hearing provides cues for action**
While one could certainly do many movement and sports skills without hearing, much information about a movement task is obtained through the auditory sense. For some activities, such as dance, sound is critical! Infants may hear sounds before birth but the ability to link sound information with that from other senses improves during childhood. Children also improve in their ability to discriminate sounds especially if they have been given the opportunity to hear many sounds and challenged to discriminate increasingly similar sounds. To use sound information in movement activities to advantage one needs to perceive many things about a sound in addition to merely "hearing" it. One sometimes should attend to one sound against a background of other noises. This ability is called auditory figure-ground perception. Also the direction from which a sound comes must be determined. Particularly important in dance and rhythmic activities is the ability to perceive rhythms.

# How Do I Get It?

Developing skills
involves use of the
laws of motion and
stability

There are many, many different motor skills, each with its own purpose. There are a few basic tasks performers attempt to do in most of the movements possible with the human body. Many times, for example, one attempts to propel an object. This is the case in kicking a soccer ball, driving a puck in ice hockey, throwing a football, striking a tennis ball, and so on. Other times one's goal is to propel the body through space. Running is this kind of skill as is a high jump and gymnastic skills. To execute these tasks well the performer should do them according to the laws of motion which dictate the most efficient ways to perform skills. In all of these a performer needs to make the body as stable as possible. There are laws or principles which suggest how to do this. A third purpose in skills is to absorb force as in catching a ball, landing from a jump, or falling on the ground! These activities are too governed by principles which dictate optimal performance of a task. There is never just one way to perform a skill. Its execution is determined by the skill goal. As discussed everyone has a differently shaped body, different strengths, and different experiences. These differences may mean one style of performing a skill is better for a particular person than another. Form and style are different aspects of a skill. Physical principles, however, generally tell one which basic movement patterns should be present in skills to produce a maximum effort. To perform optimally everyone must learn to do physical skills in accordance with the laws of motion, stability, and force absorption. The booklet on kinesiology will give more information about these principles. As a child develops, one should see the basic skills performed more and more in accordance with these laws.

Goals and body
differences may vary
skill performance

# How?

Relatively short legs
give children a higher
center of gravity

It is often important to make the body as stable as possible so that one remains upright and does not fall. At other times performers want to make their bodies *unstable* so that they can move through space as in walking or running. The terms static and dynamic are applicable. The Kinesiology booklet in the "Basic Stuff" series explains "center of gravity" and "base of support" and how they relate to a sense of equilibrium.

As already mentioned body proportions change with age. Along with these growth changes there is a change in the relative location of the center of gravity within the body. In infancy and early childhood the center of gravity for an upright position is relatively higher in the trunk than an adult's because the legs are relatively shorter. Young children first learning to walk and run widen their base of support to accomodate the difficulty they have with lateral balance. By the preschool and school years children should have little difficulty in alternately losing and regaining their balance in the forward direction, as in walking or running, while maintaining lateral balance. Hence by the school years the practical significance of the slightly higher center of gravity in young children to the maintenance of balance is probably minimal.

# How Do I Get It?

**Developmental factors and mechanical principles guide the changes in running form**

By the age of 5 most children have developed a basic running form. Refinement of the running pattern may continue through into adolescence permitting increased speed as well as locomotion along variable paths on variable surfaces. These refinements are consistent with the laws of motion; application of sound mechanical principles improves performance. It is known that for every action there is an equal and opposite reaction. When runners push against the ground with their rear leg the ground pushes back and sends the runner into the "flight" phase of the run. One of the developmental trends in running is an increase in the extension of the pushing leg reflecting an optimal force application. The amount of time the runner is in "flight" also increases with age partly because the legs are longer as a result of this optimal force.

It is also known from the laws of motion that a shorter limb is easier to move than a longer one. After the propelling leg in running pushes off the ground it is bent to be brought forward more easily. As children mature there is an increase in the bend of the leg to bring the heel close to the buttocks as the leg is swung forward. Older children bring their swing leg forward more efficiently. They are also raising the height of their knee at the end of the leg swing. These actions help increase the length of the running stride and thus running speed as the child develops a more mature running form (see Figures 3-1 and 3-2). When the swing leg straightens, the foot lands on the ground under the center of gravity and the knee will slightly bend to absorb the force of landing.

One can run forward more efficiently if the body-produced forces are directed in the direction of the run rather than to the side or unnecessarily upward. As the running form matures there is less sideward and upward movement; energy for movement is used in the desired direction. A slight forward lean of the trunk is maintained in a mature pattern.

At the early stages of running, jumping, hopping, or other locomotor movement children have a tendency to carry their arms high and stiff with little movement to enhance balance. With maturing form the action of the arms will follow the law of "action/reaction." As the right leg moves back the right arm moves forward in reaction. The left leg is forward at this time but the left arm has moved back in reaction. The arms are bent at the elbows at about a right angle following the law which says a shorter limb moves more easily than a larger one.

Other locomotor skills are learned soon after running. Some children may be able to gallop with the preferred foot forward as early as two years. Later a sideward slide is added. A skip may be performed by some children at 4 years of age while others may not perfect skipping until 7 years. Most of the mechanical principles we discussed for running can be found in these locomotor skills. Increased periods of flight come with maturing patterns as more force is produced by the child along the direction of motion. The arms and legs are coordinated following the law of action/reaction especially in the skip. Hopping and jumping are also locomotor movements which are enjoyable and basic to sport skills.

# How Do I Get It?

**Developmental changes consistent with the laws of motion improve jumping performance**

At two years of age most children can jump vertically upward or downward from a small height onto one foot. Thereafter children progressively attempt more difficult jumps as well as hopping which is usually performed for the first time at 3 or 4 years. Jumps which would be progressively more

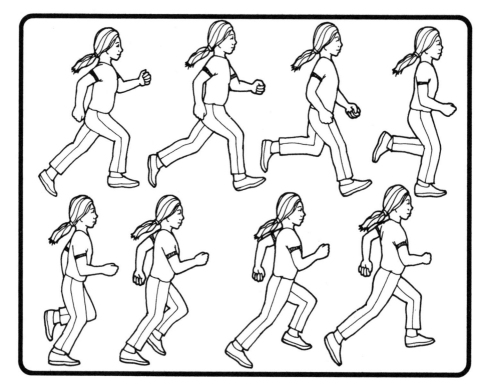

**Figure 3-1.** This five-year-old coordinates her arm and leg action. As the right leg moves back the right arm moves forward in reaction. The range of motion of the arms and legs is limited, however. Notice the limited bend in the knee of the recovery leg and the limited height of the knee. This keeps the length of the running stride and therefore the running speed below maximum.

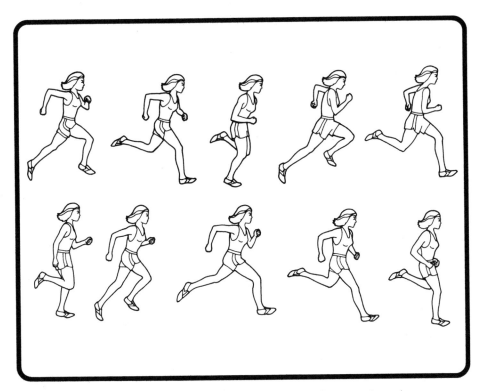

**Figure 3-2.** Notice that this runner, showing mature form in the sprint, has a long stride. The recovery leg is maximally bent and the recovery knee is high. The support leg extends fully to propel the runner forward and upward.

difficult are: a jump up with two feet to two feet; a jump down with one foot to two then two feet to two feet; a run-and-leap; a two-foot jump forward; a jump over an object; rhythmic hopping. By school age jumping ability is usually assessed by the distance jumped in the standing broad jump or the vertical jump rather than the type of jump mastered. Typically, steady improvements in jumping distance or height can be observed at successive ages. Hopping requires greater strength and balance develops later.

While an increase in strength certainly plays a role in improved jumping performance, developmental changes in jumping form consistent with the laws of motion are also occurring. At an early age the vertical jump of a child is characterized by a very small preparatory crouch, a slight forward lean at take-off and some forward movement, a high, stiff arm position or a "wing" arm position, and a quick bending of the hips and knees to tuck the legs under the body. As the movement pattern for the vertical jump becomes more mature the preliminary crouch will increase, the arms will be used for lift, the legs will extend at take-off, and the trunk will extend at the height of the jump. In the preparatory crouch the hips, knees, and ankles are all bent. The arms begin the jump with a powerful lift, then the hips, knees, and ankles extend. The body is straight until the ankles, knees, and hips bend to absorb the force of landing (see Figures 3-3 and 3-4). The exact form to be used for jumping often depends on the goal of the jump for both children and adults. For example the arm position in a child's jump would be quite different if the child were told to "jump as high as possible" rather than "jump and reach" for an object placed overhead. The first instruction may bring out little use of the arms while the second may bring a mature pattern of the arms moving upward, one arm reaching for the object and the other swinging down in opposition.

The standing long jump may first appear with a form identical to that of the vertical jump. There is increasingly more horizontal distance covered as the pattern of the jump matures. The preliminary crouch increases as does the forward swing of the arms. The jumper takes off more horizontally with the body having fully extended at take-off. During the jump the hips bend so that the thigh is nearly horizontal at landing.

These changes in the jump reflect applications of sound mechanical principles. For example it is known that a body tends to remain at rest unless force is applied to it. More speed can be gained by increasing the distance over which a force is

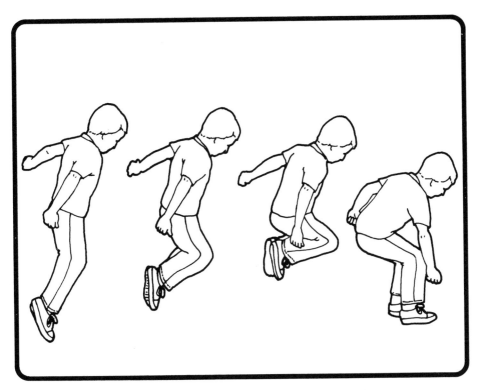

**Figure 3-3.** The vertical jump of this boy has several characteristics of immature form. The legs are quickly bent after take-off and tucked under the body rather than extended. The arms are not used for lift but held in a "winging" position, and there is some forward as well as upward movement.

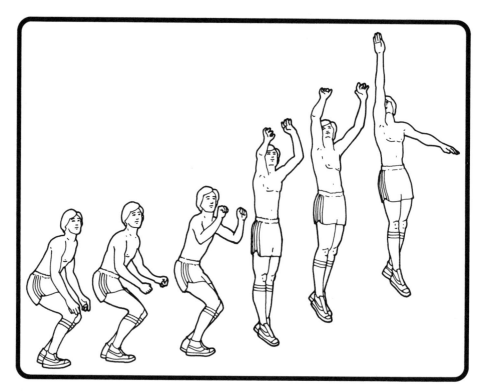

**Figure 3-4.** In the mature vertical jump-and-reach, there is a deep preparatory crouch and extension of the hips, knees, and ankles. The arms are used first for lift, then one arm reaches for the object while the other arm swings down in opposition.

applied. By crouching deeply before a jump one can increase the distance over which muscle force is exerted. The direction of a jump is the result of the amount of direction of the forces applied. If performers want to jump up they need to direct their muscular force upward. If they need to jump forward for distance most of the muscular force should be directed in the horizontal direction.

Efficient performance on tasks like jumping are usually a result of applying muscular force in steps with each new force applied as the previous one ends. In the jump the performer ideally should have arm action followed by the beginning of hip extension, then knee extension, and finally ankle extension. Poor performers begin these movements at the same time rather than successively. The law of action and reaction is also seen in jumping. The flight is a result of pushing against the ground and having it push back. The bend at the hip during the flight of a mature jumper is a reaction to the forward movement of the trunk.

# How Do I Get It?

Learning to absorb force is necessary for safe participation

Performers sometimes fall when playing hard. In some sports like judo or wrestling, falling is a part of the sport. It is also necessary to catch hard balls or to deflect fast moving balls or pucks, as a part of many games and sports. In all of these cases the moving body or the moving object has *force*. One needn't get hurt in these activities if one knows how to *absorb* this force properly. The Kinesiology booklet explains in detail how to properly absorb force. Basically it is easier to absorb force if one increases the *area* of impact and the *distance* over which the force is absorbed. Young performers sometimes need instruction in exactly what movements will increase the impact area or the distance.

When catching, many young children react by turning their head away or closing their eyes. This is probably the result of being hit in the face with throws too difficult for young children to catch. In early attempts to catch children scoop the ball into their arms and trap it against their bodies. Gradually an effort is made to contact the ball with the hands. In mature catching the arms are bent in preparation to "give" with the catch. The arms adjust to move the hands to the ball and the hands close on the ball with contact (see Figures 3-5 and 3-6).

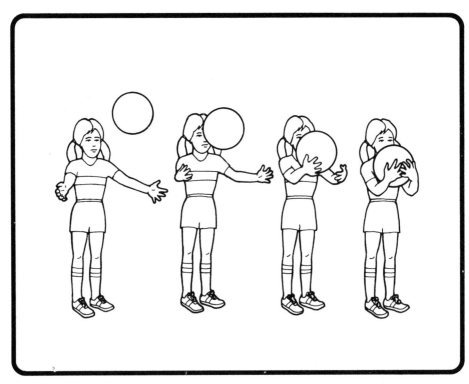

**Figure 3-5.** This young girl extends her arms and spreads her fingers as the ball approaches. She uses a clapping motion to contact the ball then traps it against her chest.

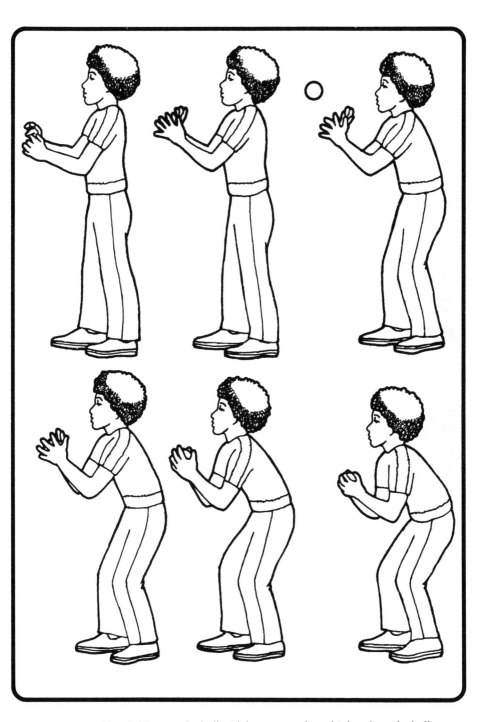

**Figure 3-6.** The older child awaits the ball with bent arms, closes his hands on the ball, and ''gives'' with the catch.

# How Do I Get It?

Catching and striking
require complex
perceptual judgments
Part of the challenge in catching is predicting where the ball will be and when it will be there so that the hands can be positioned properly. The same is true of striking skills wherein the striking implement must arrive at the proper place at the proper time. So catching and striking require complex perceptual judgments, predictions based on the perceptual information, as well as a plan for executing the movement itself. Characteristics of the task can make the perceptual judgments harder or easier. For example, a ball approaching in a high trajectory is more difficult to judge than a flat one. A small ball requires a more accurate prediction than a large one, and so on. Because these complex perceptual judgments are involved in catching and striking, young children typically execute ballistic skills like throwing and stationary kicking better than they catch or strike. Repeated practice with a variety of perceptual conditions is required for improved judgment.

# How Do I Get It?

Perfection of form aids
in increasing distance
Many of the sport and recreational activities one can enjoy with other people throughout life require throwing, kicking, or striking skills. These skills have many mechanical factors in common since the purpose of all these tasks is to give an object, usually a ball, speed. More is known about the throwing form of children than their striking or kicking form. Some of the developmental changes in throwing, however, may be similar to those in kicking and striking. The developmental changes in throwing will be examined first and then one may look for similarities in striking and kicking. Because throwing is such a complicated skill it can be broken down into parts.

The trunk action of young throwers changes as their throwing patterns mature. Initially there is no action of the trunk in throwing; only the arm is active. Children then begin to bend forward at the waist with the throw. If a strong throw is attempted they may first bend back then forward. In becoming more mature in their throw children will twist their upper spine back then forward with the throw. Later rotation of the hips back then forward in unison with the upper spine is added. Eventually a tipping of the trunk to the side away from the throwing arm may appear. This allows for a true *overarm* throw. In the most mature form of the throw this tipping of the trunk remains but the hips begin to rotate forward before the upper spine. The upper body, in fact, may still be twisting to the back.

These developmental changes in trunk action for the overarm throw are similar to those for the sidearm throw, one-handed sidearm striking, and two-handed sidearm striking. In kicking as form matures there is more hip rotation backward as the leg swings back and rotation forward with the kick. All of these actions allow the distance over which muscle force is applied to the ball to be increased. The sequential action of the trunk is also consistent with the mechanical principle discussed earlier wherein a maximal skill has forces applied in steps.

**Growth and development of trunk and arms improves throwing capability**

Mature tasks which propel an object also have a common characteristic called "opening up." In the throw a mature performer is typically taking a step forward while the hand and ball are still moving to the back. Even during trunk rotation forward the ball and hand are still lagging back. This characteristic is also based on the principle of applying forces in steps with each new force applied as the previous force is making its greatest contribution to giving the ball speed.

The arm action in the throw, like trunk action, appears to develop in stages as children become more proficient. Initially the upper arm moves forward above or below horizontal. If one looks at a young child throwing, the elbow is either pointing up or down. In more mature steps, however, the upper arm will come forward at a right angle with the trunk, horizontally in line with the shoulders. This forward movement is not simultaneous though with trunk rotation-forward in the mature throw. The elbow will be in front by the time the trunk has rotated forward but the upper arm will be behind the trunk. After the trunk has rotated forward to face the target the upper arm will come forward.

If the elbow of a beginning thrower is observed it will be seen that it is completely bent before the throwing movement or bends as the arm is coming forward. As the thrower's form develops the elbow will be only partially bent before the arm moves or as it begins to move (see Figures 3-7 and 3-8). This bend remains until the elbow is straightened with the throw. In the most advanced throwing form the elbow will be held at roughly a right angle from the end of the backswing until it straightens with the throw.

The position of the upper arm and elbow naturally affects the position of the lower arm as does the rotation of the upper arm at the shoulder. Initially the lower arm comes forward

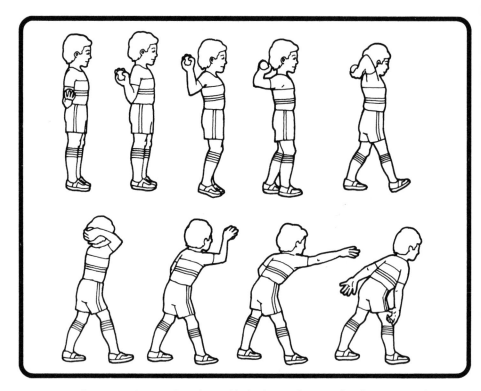

**Figure 3-7.** The young thrower here has added a forward step to his throw to produce additional force but the step is with the same side, rather than opposite leg. Note also the bend in the throwing arm at release and limited trunk rotation.

# ERRATA

The names listed on the title pages of each book in *Basic Stuff Series I* are the revisions authors for the 1987 edition. The original (1981) author teams are as follows:

*Exercise Physiology*

Milan Svoboda, Portland State University, Oregon
Maxine Thomas, Portland State University, Oregon
Donna Bergmann, Beaverton School District, Beaverton, Oregon
George Rochat, Catlin Gabel School, Portland, Oregon

*Kinesiology*

Geraldine Greenlee, Illinois State University, Normal
Helen Heitmann, University of Illinois, Chicago
Barbara Cothren, Illinois Wesleyan University, Bloomington
Dolores Hellweg, Illinois State University, Normal

*Motor Learning*

Anne Rothstein, Herbert Lehman College, City University of New York
Linda Catelli, Queens College, City University of New York
Patt Dodds, University of Massachusetts, Amherst
Joan Manahan, Teaneck Public Schools, Teaneck, New Jersey

*Psycho-Social Aspects of Physical Education*

Carole Oglesby, Temple University, Philadelphia
Lee A. Bell, State University of New York, New Paltz
Patricia S. Griffin, University of Massachusetts, Amherst

*Humanities in Physical Education*

Ginny Studer, State University of New York, Brockport
Mary E. Kazlusky, Cortland, New York
Susan Gardner, Rome Free Academy, Rome, New York
Diane Guinan, Washington College, Chestertown, Maryland

*Motor Development*

Kathleen Haywood, University of Missouri, St. Louis
Thomas Loughery, University of Missouri, St. Louis
Michael Imergoot, Ferguson-Florissant School District, St. Louis County, Missouri
Karen Wilson, Ferguson-Florissant School District, St. Louis County, Missouri

In addition, page 5 of each of the *Series I* books lists the revision committee for the 1987 edition of *Series II*; the original Basic Stuff editorial committee for the 1981 edition included the following:

Marian E. Kneer, Editor, University of Illinois, Chicago
Linda L. Bain, University of Houston, Texas
Norma J. Carr, State University of New York, Cortland
Don Hellison, Portland State University, Oregon
Mary Kazlusky, Cortland, New York
Barbara Lockhart, University of Iowa, Iowa City
Jack Razor, University of Georgia, Athens
Sandra Wilbur, Cape May Beach, New Jersey

AAHPERD wishes to recognize the important contributions of the original writers and editors.

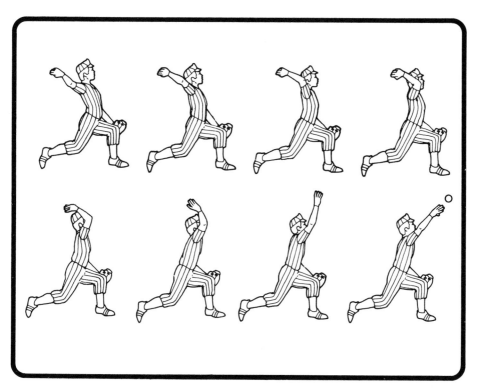

**Figure 3-8.** Notice the extension of the throwing arm at release of the ball by this baseball pitcher pictured right to left. The hips have already rotated forward but even as the upper trunk is rotating forward the arm and hand have lagged back so that force will be applied to the ball in steps.

with the upper arm until in the most mature action the lower arm will remain back until the upper trunk has rotated forward.

It is known from the laws of motion that one can increase the speed of the hand (or an object in the hand) by increasing the length of the arm. Similarly the foot can impart more speed to a kicked ball by increasing the leg length. Obviously the limbs are a fixed length at any given time but one can maximize the speed of the object being propelled by having the arm or leg nearly straight at release or contact with the ball. At the final moment of contact or release all of the muscle forces have been applied and the arm or leg is nearly straight to give the object high speed (see Figures 3-9 and 3-10), even though force is applied in steps.

Young children tend to primarily throw with their arm. They use little trunk action and may not move their feet. When they do begin to take a step with the throw it may be the foot on the same side as the throwing hand. Eventually they should step with the opposite foot. The step forward is important in striking and kicking skills as well as throwing. It increases the distance over which force can be applied to the object propelled.

# How Do I Get It?

**Improved mechanical efficiency and increased size contribute to quantitative improvements in skill**

Improvements in the mechanical efficiency of skill performance bring about improvements in quantitative measures of skill performance. These quantitative measures include the *speed* of movement, the *distance* of movement, and the *accuracy* of movement. Increased physical size through growth also results in quantitative improvements. If young children 2 to 7 years of age make the mechanical refinements discussed earlier for each of the mechanical skills, preadolescence and adolescence are subsequently periods of steady improvement in speed, distance, and accuracy.

**Running speed, and jumping and throwing distance improve steadily**

Running ability is often measured by one's speed over a short distance (often 30 yards) or in an agility run. Children typically improve from a speed of just under 4 yards per second at age 4 to approximately 6 yards per second at age 12 (Espenschade & Eckert, 1980). Boys attain a speed of 7 yards per second by age 17 but girls tend to level off. Speed in an agility run also improves steadily from 5 to 18 years of age but girls do not attain the speeds achieved by boys in adolescence.

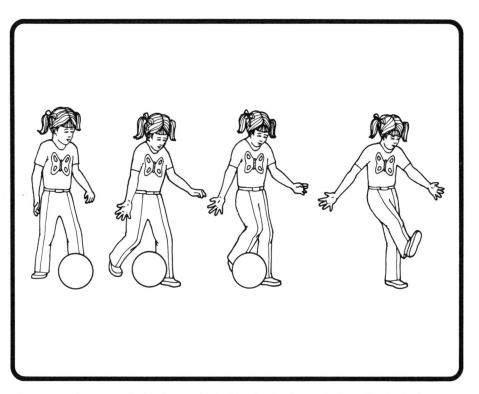

**Figure 3-9.** This young kicker brings the kicking leg back to gain force for the kick but notice that the leg is bent at the time of contact with the ball.

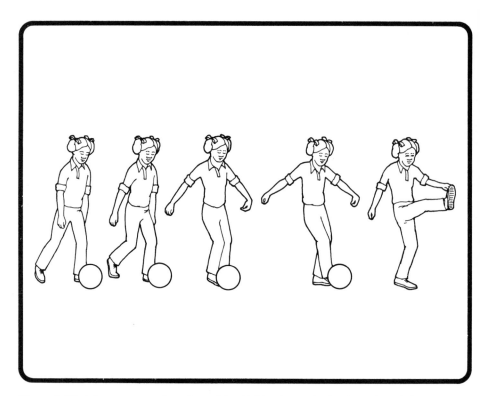

**Figure 3-10.** A larger range of motion of the kicking leg and a backward trunk lean characterize the more mature kicking form of this child.

Improved performance is demonstrated, too, in horizontal and vertical jumping distance. Between 5 and 11 years, for example, children increase their horizontal jump distance from approximately 33 inches to 60 inches. Boys improve steadily to approximately 90 inches by age 17 but girls plateau in adolescence.

Throwing distance reflects differences in boys' and girls' performance from even young ages. Boys increase their distance from approximately 24 feet to 153 feet between 5 and 17 years, but girls improve from 14.5 feet to approximately 75 feet. Children also increase their throwing speed.

Quantitative measures of skill performance can reflect factors in addition to mechanical efficiency and body size. For example, body composition and strength level affect performance. So, too, do the instructions given children in a performance test.

Even social factors influence performance and this might in part account for girls' poorer quantitative performance compared to boys. In the past it was often considered socially unacceptable for adolescent girls and women to give an all-out effort in a skill test, particularly if this resulted in outscoring boys or men. This attitude may have changed somewhat in recent years but such well-established attitudes do not change rapidly. There is evidence in more recent studies of running speed and jumping distance that adolescent girls as a group are improving their performance through adolescence. Of course, size differences also contribute to differences in quantitative performance.

# How Do I Get It?

**In skilled performance, basic skills must be combined and adapted to task demands**

To achieve skilled levels of performance, children must learn to combine or link skills. For example, a young basketball player must learn to dribble on the run, jump, and shoot the ball off the backboard for a layup. Children must also learn to adapt skill execution to a variety of situations. The same young basketball player must learn to execute the layup if there is an opponent alongside, other opponents to dribble around and between, and so on.

Teachers can be of great help to children in combining and adapting skills. This assistance is given by teachers when they plan various drill and practice situations. The conditions should initially be simple, and then increased in complexity as children demonstrate their ability to meet task demands.

The complexity of a practice condition can be increased by changing the speed or trajectory of a ball, changing the size of a ball or the size and distance of the field, court, basket, etc., complicating the path taken (as in zigzag dribbling), adding defensive players, and so on.

**Qualitative and quantitative improvements are related**

Many times challenging children to improve their quantitative performance (as "throw farther") will elicit an improvement in mechanical efficiency. That is, the child "discovers" the *way* to make the ball travel farther, for example. Mechanical improvements then lead to further quantitative improvements. Hence, movement pattern, or qualitative, improvements and quantitative advancements go hand-in-hand. Teachers might elicit an improvement by a direct teaching cue (as saying "take a step with your left foot" or "take a longer step") or designing a practice situation that challenges children to improve. This emphasizes the importance of challenging all children to reach higher levels. If girls in particular are not expected to perform at a high level and therefore not challenged to do so, they will not discover the ways to actually perform well.

# How Do I Get It?

**Practice makes perfect (or at least better)**

Changes in the form of many skills have been examined. These changes increase skill performance but usually for speed rather than accuracy. It has been noted that applying muscle forces in the direction one desires to move or propel an object is the most efficient way to perform the skill. Beyond this, practice is necessary to increase accuracy. The best ways to practice are discussed in the Motor Learning booklet.

**Skills improve when the body is ready and with supervised practice**

Each person will acquire improvements in movement patterns at different ages. Sometimes one part of the pattern, say, the trunk action, will be fairly mature while another, maybe the arm action, is at a beginning level. Typically children at two years of age are just beginning to attempt these basic skills. During the next five years their movement patterns improve in form so that by age seven their basic skills resemble those of an adult. Improvement isn't automatic though. There are many adults who have immature characteristics in their performance. This is why it is helpful for a child to have a teacher observe performance. The teacher can suggest changes or new ways a skill may be practiced to develop a mature motor pattern. Some improvements in skill have to wait until the body is also ready. Sometimes it is necessary to wait until one grows taller. At other times, it may be found that becoming stronger will help performance. One may have to exercise to increase strength, flexibility, or endurance and find that this too will help. It is possible for everyone to improve and be successful at motor skills and to enjoy them. One may not be the best at every skill but with the help of teachers and hard work improvement can be made. The phylogenetic skills of running, jumping, and other forms of locomotion appear to depend more upon neuromuscular maturation and experience than do the ontogenetic skills of catching, throwing, and kicking. These latter appear to respond more to teaching suggestions than do the former.

# psycho-social

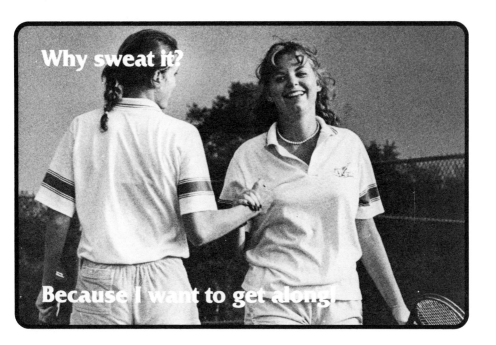

Why sweat it?

Because I want to get along!

## What Have You Got To Help Me?

One of the most important contributions that sport and games can make for a person is to provide an outlet for social interaction and a showcase for personal competence. The booklet *Psycho-Social Aspects of Physical Education* in the "Basic Stuff" series should be consulted for a detailed understanding of factors related to "getting along" through involvement in meaningful movement experiences.

**Sports and games allow opportunities to evaluate personal attributes**

Getting along with others begins by accepting the personal self and physical capabilities and then confidently relating to others. Participation in sports and games allows a person opportunities to evaluate his personal skills as well as those of his peers. In addition play permits testing a variety of

**Play permits testing of a variety of social behaviors** behaviors in terms of their social acceptance. When a person can accept himself he can then reach out to others by sharing, caring, and helping. Such behavior may be confidently given if a person's self-image and self-concept is healthy. Success and enjoyment of meaningful physical activities may contribute significantly to the development of social interaction. Conversely, failure experiences make an equally negative impact. Consequently engaging in physical activities must be realistically pursued since it has been pointed out earlier that performance will be affected by the stage of growth and degree of motor development.

Finally the cathartic effect achieved through physical activity may result in an overall feeling of goodness and that feeling enables a person to accept and appreciate the performance of others. Furthermore successful participation in physical activities increases self-confidence and the likelihood of being accepted and appreciated by others.

# How Do I Get It?

**Play should be with those of similiar abilities** Ability to "get along" may be increased or improved by applying knowledge about growth and motor development when planning or engaging in physical activity. Since self-acceptance and other acceptance is important to developing healthy social interaction it is vital that a reasonable opportunity exists for successful participation. Consequently selecting appropriate activities for the person's growth and motor development is imperative. The activity skill requirements should be within range of the normal growth and motor development capabilities of the performers. Similiarly if the game or sport is competitively played the participants should be similiar with their development stage.

**Personal goal setting fosters self and other acceptance** Setting achievable goals in terms of growth and motor development of the participant will foster self and other esteem for all participants. Heavy commitment to group goals should be avoided in favor of personal goal setting. Finally every performer should position the values of playing, winning, and personal accomplishment in perspective of the time, place, and overall importance to human well-being.

# coping

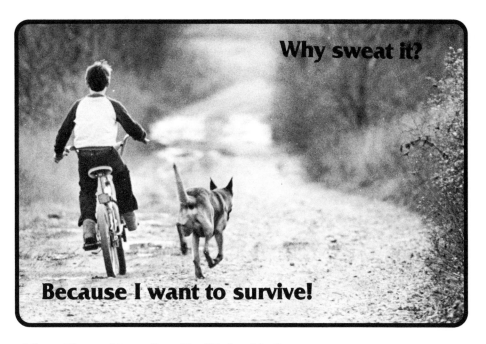

Why sweat it?

Because I want to survive!

## What Have You Got To Help Me?

At every stage of physical development, from infancy through old age, the way a person looks and moves greatly influences relationships with others. Given society's tendency to judge on appearance and skill, the person whose physical appearance or movement patterns are unpleasant will sometimes be ridiculed or excluded from social activities.

Through an understanding of growth patterns and efficient movement patterns, a person can develop a sense of self-acceptance based on personal potentials and limitations. Because certain aspects of personal appearance are genetically determined, a person must learn to accept those factors that are fixed, such as height and facial features. Those factors that can change to improve appearance, such as body alignment, body composition and development of musculature, can be included in a program of self improvement.

For example, the adolescent girl who develops improper body alignment because she is self-conscious about being the tallest in the class should understand that her growth rate is much faster than most and, in time, other classmates might surpass her. Similarly, a person who develops slowly in motor skill should realize that slow progress does not mean a lifetime of poor skill. Quantitative measures of performance are particularly subject to physical size. Late maturers are likely to improve in speed and distance when their body size increases with growth. A person can continue to practice and make diligent efforts to develop mature movement patterns. Combinations of skills and various adaptations of skill to environmental conditions can also be learned.

Thus, the person can identify those activities in which efficient movement patterns have not been mastered and begin a program leading to personal improvement. These changes can help one cope with one's self and others as well as survive socially in spite of, or because of, one's physical well-being and motor development.

**Goals need to be realistic**

A necessary first step in this change process is to set realistic and attainable goals and in doing so one needs to be aware of individual needs and capabilities. Goals are easier to attain if one is motivated and interested in that area or activity. To determine a person's motivation level in a certain activity it is necessary to determine whether or not participation in that particular activity would meet any of the person's needs. If motivation is lacking, a high goal expectation in that activity will not exist. If motivation is strong the person probably will be able to set a relatively high goal.

As one matures the importance of individual goal setting and attainment increases and the importance of group acceptance decreases. Therefore it is possible to survive in any task if one can accept how he performs a task in relation to how others perform the task or how he performed the task earlier. This should lead to the development of a realistic self-concept based on individual goal attainment.

**Improvement is possible but gradual**

An important phase of the coping and surviving process is the personal improvement phase. Personal improvement in motor tasks and appearance is readily evident in the development and maturation process. For example an infant has little early success in learning to walk but gradually through persistent practice the motor act of walking is mastered. Many changes in motor performance and appearance are possible and constant improvement should be a goal. Such improvement and changes may lead to a higher level of self and peer acceptance. As one achieves success in the process of improvement one can more accurately develop goals for further improvement.

It will be difficult to institute a personal improvement program without the assistance of others. No problem should be considered to be too great or too embarrassing to share with others. When a student asks for help physical education and health teachers know which behaviors need to be changed to bring about improvement in physical ability and appearance factors. Also the teachers will be able to determine which appearance factors may be changed and which may not be changed. These teachers should be able to assist in the goal setting process and in the construction of self-improvement programs. If necessary they may refer one to other professionals in the school and in outside agencies who may be able to assist in the improvement process. Also much personal assistance may be given by parents, classmates, and friends.

There are many factors that interact to determine the amount of satisfaction one has about personal appearance, participation in physical activities, and relations with others. Many times a person does not consider what effect certain body factors and physical ability factors have on their level of self-concept and acceptance by others. As each comes to understand the relationship between these factors and their level of self-fulfillment and satisfaction they will better be able to set goals that are realistic and attainable.

**Satisfaction results from attaining goals**

It is difficult in a school setting to experience the freedom necessary to set goals and determine levels of satisfaction that should result from participation in physical activity. By its nature the school imposes certain situational restraints such as teacher-set expectations for all students and grading procedures that demand certain attainment levels. For example all students in a class or grade level are expected to achieve a specific level of success in a particular activity. Seldom is the level of physical development considered in designing that outcome. Therefore students who greatly differ from the norm in developmental factors, body factors, or physical ability level may find the expected outcome either to be very easy or nearly impossible to achieve.

Participation in physical activity should be undertaken to accomplish a wide variety of self-fulfillment goals. Broad areas of student purposes for participation as well as specific student purposes are described by Jewett and Mullan.* Re-

*Jewett, A. E.; and Mullan, M. R. *Curriculum Design: Purposes and Processes in Physical Education Teaching-Learning*. Washington, DC: AAHPER, 1977.

gardless of the specific goal or purpose that motivates people of all ages to participate, a feeling of accomplishment satisfaction or self-fulfillment is a desirable outcome. Many physical, psychological, social, and emotional factors are present in most participation settings and situations that greatly affect the negative or positive feelings resulting from participation.

To help one understand himself and his relations with others in activity settings it may be helpful to determine one's purposes for participation, the goals one sets, and the outcome one expects to achieve. By doing this one may begin to see that the level of aspiration needed to result in one's feeling of fulfillment may differ dramatically from others in the same activity setting. While some may feel that success is measured only in quantifiable terms such as placing near the top in that event, others may measure success in qualitative terms such as how good it felt to expend energy. As one comes to realize and accept purposes and goals for participation one may come to an understanding of himself and his relation with others.

Change is an essential ingredient in any educational experience and one should constantly see the process of change as an important factor in self-improvement programs. One should also know that previously discussed environmental factors relating to personal appearance such as body composition and body alignment, can be changed. If a student perceives that these factors limit his ability to achieve success in physical activities or to be accepted by others then teachers can encourage him to consider engaging in programs that will modify these factors.

# Where Can I Find More Information?

Corbin, C. *A Textbook of Motor Development*. 2d ed. Dubuque, IA: W. C. Brown Co., 1980.

Cratty, B. *Perceptual and Motor Development in Infants and Children*. 2d ed. Englewood Cliffs, NJ: Prentice-Hall, Inc., 1979.

Espenschade, A. S., & Eckert, H. M. (1980). *Motor development* (2nd ed.). Columbus, OH: Charles E. Merrill.

Gallahue, D. L. (1982). *Understanding motor development*. New York: John Wiley & Sons.

Haywood, K. M. (1986). *Life span motor development*. Champaign, IL: Human Kinetics.

Keogh, J., & Sugden, D. (1985). *Movement skill development*. New York: Macmillan Publishing.

Malina, R. *Growth and Development: The First Twenty Years In Man*. Minneapolis: Burgess Publishing Co., 1975.

Rarick, G. L., *Physical Activity: Human Growth and Development*. New York: Academic Press, 1973.

Ridenour, M., ed. *Motor Development Issues and Applications*. Princeton, NJ: Princeton Book Company, 1978.

Robertson, M. A., & Halverson, L. E. (1984). *Developing children—Their changing movement*. Philadelphia: Lea & Febiger.

Shephard, R. J. (1982). *Physical activity and growth:* Chicago: Year Book Medical Publishers.

Teeple, J. B.; and Wirth, J. "Updated bibliographies: Physical growth and motor development." *The Physical Educator 34:* 241-220.

Thomas, J. R. (Ed.) (1984). *Motor development during childhood and adolescence*. Minneapolis, MN: Burgess Publishing.

Williams, H. (1983). *Perceptual and motor development*. Englewood Cliffs: Prentice-Hall.

Wickstrom, R. L. (1983). *Fundamental motor patterns* (3rd ed.). Philadelphia: Lea & Febiger.

Zaichkowsky, L. E.; Zaichlowsky, L. B.; and Martinek, T. J. *Growth and Development: The Child and Physical Activity*. St. Louis: C..V. Mosby Company, 1980.